Copyright 2020

Contents

PREVIEW

Fatty liver disease is becoming increasingly common in many parts of the world, affecting about 25% of people globally.

It is linked to obesity, type 2 diabetes and other disorders characterized by insulin resistance.

What's more, if fatty liver isn't addressed, it may progress to more serious liver disease and other health problems.

FATTY LIVER DISEASE RECIPES

BREAKFAST

1. Curry Scrambled Eggs

Prep Time: 5 minutes

Cook Time: 15 minutes

Total Time: 20 minutes

Servings: 4

Ingredients

- 1 tablespoon avocado oil
- 2 cups leftover chicken breast or thighs, diced (you can substitute pre-cooked
- sausage, ham, or tofu if vegetarian)
- 1/4 onion, diced
- 1 cup mushrooms, diced
- 4 cups kale (or sub spinach or other greens work too)
- 6 eggs
- 1 tablespoon curry powder

- Salt and pepper to taste

Instructions

1. Heat a large skillet over medium heat.
2. Add in the leftover chicken and onion. Cook for about 5 minutes, stirring occasionally.
3. While the chicken is cooking, crack your eggs into a medium bowl. Whisk with a fork until the eggs are mixed well.
4. Add in the kale and mushrooms to the skillet. Cook for another 5 minutes stirring occasionally.
5. Dump in the eggs and curry powder. Mix everything together well to get the curry powder all mixed in. Cook the eggs for a few minutes until they are no longer runny and are to your desired scrambled state.
6. Season with salt and pepper to taste.
7. Serve and enjoy your breakfast...or lunch...or dinner!

2. Homemade Pumpkin Bagels

Prep Time: 10 minutes

Cook Time: 25 minutes

Total Time: 35 mintes

Servings: 8 Bagels

Ingredients

- Dry Ingredients:
- 1/3 cup coconut flour
- 3 tablespoon flaxseed meal
- 1 1/2 teaspoon pumpkin pie spice
- 1/2 teaspoon cinnamon
- Pinch of salt
- 1/2 teaspoon baking soda
- Wet Ingredients:
- 3 whole eggs
- 2 tablespoon coconut oil melted
- 1/4 cup non-dairy milk of choice (I used almond milk)

- 1/2 cup pumpkin puree

- 1 teaspoon vanilla extract

- 2 tablespoon maple syrup

- 1 teaspoon apple cider vinegar

Instructions

1. Preheat oven to 350°F and grease a donut or bagel pan.
2. In a bowl, add the dry ingredients, except for the baking soda, and mix until well combined.
3. In a separate bowl, add the wet ingredients, except for the apple cider vinegar, and mix until well combined.
4. In a small bowl, mix the apple cider vinegar and baking soda. Add this mixture to the wet ingredients.
5. Slowly add the dry mixture into the wet until well combined and the batter is smooth.
6. Pipe or spoon the batter into the prepared pan until all molds have an even amount of batter.
7. Bake for about 22-25 minutes or until a toothpick comes out clean. Remove from the oven and let sit for about 5 minutes before removing from the pan onto a cooling rack.

8. Serve and enjoy! Can be topped with ghee, nut butter, or even a chocolate spread.

3. Oatmeal Raspberry Applesauce Muffins

Prep Time: 10 minutes

Cook Time: 15 minutes

Total Time: 25 minutes

Servings: 12

Ingredients

- cooking spray (I use coconut oil spray)
- 1 1/3 cups whole wheat pastry flour
- 3/4 cups rolled oats
- 1 teaspoon baking powder
- 1/2 teaspoon baking soda
- 3/4 teaspoon cinnamon
- 1/4 teaspoon salt
- 1 heaping cup unsweetened natural applesauce
- 1 teaspoon coconut oil
- 1/4 cup organic honey
- 1 egg (slightly beaten)
- 1/2 cup unsweetened vanilla almond milk
- 1 1/4 cup raspberries
- 3/4 cup unsweetened shredded coconut

Instructions

1. Preheat oven to 375 degrees F.

2. Line 12-cup muffin tin with liners and coat the inside of them with cooking spray.

3. In a large bowl combine flour, oats, baking powder, baking soda, cinnamon and salt. Set aside.

4. In a medium bowl combine applesauce, coconut oil, honey, egg, and almond milk.

5. Add wet ingredients to dry ingredients and stir until just combined, being careful not to over mix. The batter will be slightly lumpy. Gently fold in the raspberries.

6. Scoop batter into muffin tin.

7. Bake muffins for 15 minutes or until toothpick inserted into center comes out with just a few crumbs attached.

4. Low Carb Egg Muffins

Prep Time: 10 Minutes

Cook Time: 20 Minutes

Servings: 12

INGREDIENTS

- 7 eggs

- 3/4 cup chopped bell peppers

- 3/4 cup cooked ground beef

- 3/4 cup shredded pepper jack cheese

- 1/4 teaspoon chili powder

- 1/4 teaspoon paprika

- Pinch of salt

Instructions

1. Preheat oven to 350 degrees.

2. Crack eggs into a bowl and whisk.

3. Add all additional ingredients into the bowl, but keep 1/2 cup worth of the pepper jack cheese on the side.

4. Line a muffin tin with parchment paper cups.

5. Fill the parchment cups and sprinkle the additional 1/2 cup worth of shredded cheese on top of the egg cups.

6. Bake for 20-25 min.

5. Mixed Mushroom Rice with Toasted Sesame Oil Sauce

Prep Time: 10 minutes

Cook Time: 15 minutes

Servings: 3

Ingredients

- 8 ounces of mixed mushrooms (e.g., maitake, shitake, oyster, baby bella,
- enoki/washed, dried and roughly chopped)
- 12 garlic cloves (thinly sliced)
- 3 tablespoon extra virgin olive oil
- 1 heat of romaine lettuce (washed, dried and roughly chopped)
- 2 cups of cooked brown rice
- 4 tablespoon toasted sesame oil
- 4 teaspoon soy sauce
- 1/4 teaspoon sea salt
- ground pepper to taste
- 2 eggs (cooked)

Instructions

1. Sautee garlic with olive oil until soft.

2. Add mushrooms and sautee until cooked through, about 5-8 minutes, set aside.

3. Prepare sauce by mixing toasted sesame oil, soy sauce, sea salt and a pinch of ground pepper.

4. In a two bowls, evenly layer romaine lettuce, cooked rice, mushrooms.

5. Top each bowl with sunny side up eggs and sauce.

6. Mix and enjoy!

6. Asparagus and Feta Frittata
Prep Time: 10 Minutes

Cook Time: 45 Minutes

Servings: 6

Ingredients

- 8 eggs

- 1/2 cup half-and-half (use coconut milk for dairy-free)

- 1/2 cup diced yellow onion

- 3 garlic cloves, minced

- 2 tablespoons olive oil

- 2 teaspoons salt

- 1/4 teaspoon black pepper

- 1 teaspoon garlic powder

- 6 ounces feta cheese

- 1 pound fresh asparagus

Instructions

1. Preheat oven to 400 degrees F.

2. Chop ends off washed asparagus. Cut 1/3 of the asparagus into bite-sized pieces, leaving the rest whole. With the whole asparagus, toss with olive oil, salt, and pepper, and set aside.

3. Stovetop, turn a pan onto medium heat and add olive oil once warmed.

4. Add diced yellow onion, minced garlic, chopped asparagus, and a pinch of salt to the pan, stirring and cooking for approximately 5 minutes.

5. In a large bowl, crack eggs and whisk well.

6. Add half-and-half, salt, pepper, garlic powder, and almost all of the feta to the bowl. Set aside remaining feta.

7. In a 9×9 oven-safe square or round baking dish, add the asparagus-onion-garlic mixture to the bottom and spread evenly around the dish.

8. Pour the egg-milk-cheese mix over the veggies and spread evenly.

9. Bake for about 15 minutes, or until eggs are somewhat set, remove from oven, and add the asparagus spears on top of the frittata in a line.

10. If the asparagus start to sink, cook the frittata for a few more minutes before adding.

11. Finish baking for about 15-25 more minutes.

12. Check doneness by inserting a toothpick into the frittata. If there is no residue (and no jiggly eggs), it is done.

13. Serve warm and top with remaining feta cheese and cracked black pepper.

Prep Time: 15 minutes

Cook Time: 30 minutes

Servings: 6

Ingredients

- Crust Ingredients

- 2 cups almond flour
- 1/2 teaspoon salt
- 2 tablespoons coconut oil
- 1 large egg
- Filling Ingredients

- 1 cup ricotta cheese
- 2 cups Gruyere cheese, shredded
- 16-20 asparagus stalks, steamed (I used small cut ones)
- 1 tablespoon of olive oil
- salt and pepper

Instructions

1. In a mixer, blend all of the crust ingredients together in a mixer until well combined into a dough.
2. Roll out dough on to a cooking pan lined with parchment paper (makes it easier to take the crust off the pan when finished)
3. Preheat oven to 325 F and bake the crust for around 10 minutes. Then take out the crust to put on the toppings.
4. Spread the ricotta cheese over the whole crust surface.
5. Then cover all of the ricotta with the shredded gruyere cheese (as much cheese as you like)
6. Steam the asparagus then plunge them into ice cold water for a few seconds. Pat dry and toss in the olive oil and season with salt and pepper.
7. Next, layer the steamed asparagus stalks in a row right next to each other.
8. Finally, place the crust back into the oven for around 10-15 more minutes so that all the cheese as melted, the asparagus has darkened with some char, and the crust is golden.
9. Take it out, cut it up and serve

8. Island Lime Collagen Colada Smoothie

Prep Time: 5 minutes

Cook Time: N/A

Servings: 2

Ingredients

- 1 cup cashew milk (or milk of choice)
- 1 cup cold water
- 1 lime, cut into ⅛'s
- ½ frozen banana
- ¼ cup shredded coconut, unsweetened
- ¼ cup macadamia nuts, unsalted
- ¼ cup frozen pineapple
- zest and juice of additional lime
- 1 scoop Further Food Premium Marine Collagen
- 1 to 2 cups ice

Instructions

1. Place cashew milk, water and lime segments into blender and pulse 4-5 times to coarsely chop but not completely pulverize. Strain through fine mesh sieve

into a clean bowl, rinse blender out and pour "lime infused" milk back into it.

2. Add remaining ingredients and blend until the consistency you want is reached.

3. Add as much or little ice as you like. More ice will give you a thicker consistency, possibly requiring a straw! Whereas less ice will make it more "sip-able" ~~ either way, find a great spot to take a few minutes for yourself and escape away for a few minutes to the islands!

Prep Time: 15 mins

Cook Time: 20 mins

Servings: 4

Ingredients

- 1 pound zucchini (ends cut off and grated)

- 1 large egg (beaten)

- ½ cup almond flour

- 2 tablespoons golden flax meal

- 1 teaspoon sea salt

- 2 cloves garlic (minced)

- 1-2 tablespoons olive oil (or oil of your choice)

- pepper to taste

Instructions

1. Place grated zucchini in a colander over the sink. Add salt and gently toss to combine; let sit for 10 minutes.

Using a clean dish towel or cheesecloth, drain zucchini completely.

2. Mix together all ingredients with the zucchini (except oil) in a medium size mixing bowl.

3. Preheat a cast iron pan over medium heat. Pour in just enough oil to lightly coat the bottom.

4. Place latkes in 1-tablespoon-sized pieces into the pan, taking care not to overcrowd the pan. Cook for about 2 minutes or until the latkes begin to set up and the bottom is golden brown. Turn over and cook another 1-2 minutes or until golden. Remove from the pan and place on paper towels to drain excess oil.

5. Serve immediately while latkes are at their crispiest.

10. Immune-Boosting Blueberry Elderberry Jam

Prep Time: N/A

Cook Time: 20 Minutes

Servings: 4 Cups

Ingredients

- 4 cups frozen blueberries, thawed; or fresh blueberries, washed

- ½ cup filtered water

- 2 tablespoons fresh lemon juice

- 2 tablespoons Further Food Elderberry Soothing Syrup

- 3 teaspoons sugar-free pectin or Further Food Gelatin
- 2 cups monk fruit sweetener (or low carb sweetener of choice)

Instructions

1. Bring berries, water, and juice to a boil.

2. Remove one cup of jam mixture from heat, add pectin and monk fruit (optional), and stir until smooth.

3. Return blended ingredients to pot and bring to a boil once again. Reduce heat slightly and keep stirring for 10 minutes.

4. Remove pot from heat and pour jam into canning jars or mason jars. The sugar-free pectin will harden the jam as it cools. If using gelatin, place in the refrigerator to set.

5. Refrigerate once opened.

LUNCH

11. Chipotle Turkey Burgers
Prep Time: 5 minutes

Cook Time: 25 minutes

Servings: 4

Ingredients

For the toppings:

- 4 slices bacon

- 1 tomato, sliced into thin rounds

- 1 head romaine lettuce (or other broad leaf green)

- For the burgers:

- 2 lbs ground turkey

- 1 teaspoon chipotle powder (more or less to taste)

- 1 teaspoon garlic powder

For the guacamole:

- 2 avocados, diced into chunks

- 1/8 red onion, finely diced

- 1/4 teaspoon garlic powder

- Salt and pepper, to taste

Instructions

1. Place a large cast iron pan or skillet over medium heat and cook bacon. Cook until it reaches your desired level of crispiness.
2. Remove from heat and place on a paper towel lined plate.
3. While the bacon is cooking, prep the rest of the toppings as noted, and set aside.
4. Place burger ingredients in a large mixing bowl and use your hands to combine all the ingredients.
5. Form into evenly sized patties and place on a plate. It should make ~6 patties. Cook patties in same pan as bacon over medium heat for about 6-7 minutes each side, or until turkey is cooked all the way through.
6. While the burgers are cooking, make guacamole.
7. Place avocado chunks in a bowl and add onion, garlic powder and a pinch of salt and pepper.
8. Mix together well, slightly smashing the avocado. Set aside.
9. Once burgers are done., remove from heat and serve.
10. Use lettuce for buns and top burger with guacamole, then bacon, and tomato. Enjoy!

12. Quick & Easy Cheeseburger Salad

Prep Time:15 Minutes

Cook Time :N/A

Servings: 4

Ingredients

- 4 cups mixed lettuce, chopped

- 1 lb ground beef

- Salt and pepper, to taste

- 1 cup grape tomatoes, sliced

- ½ red onion, finely chopped

- ⅓ cup cheddar cheese, grated

- Handful of dill pickles, quartered

- 2 tablespoons thousand island dressing

- For the croutons:

- 4-6 slices of your favorite bread, hamburger or hot dog buns

- Oil spray

- Salt

Instructions

1. To make the salad: Heavily season the ground beef with salt and pepper. Saute it until it's cooked all the way through. Set aside to cool.
2. In a large bowl, add the lettuce, tomatoes, red onion, pickles, cheese and ground beef after it's cooled.
3. Mix everything together. Drizzle with dressing right before you serve and top with any additional toppings
4. To make the croutons: Preheat oven to 375 degrees and line a baking sheet with parchment paper.
5. Cut the bread into 1 inch cubes and place them in a bowl. Spray the pieces with your oil spray until they're completely coated.
6. Sprinkle these pieces with salt and any other spices to your liking. Mix everything together and pour onto your prepared baking sheet.
7. Bake for 10 minutes or until the croutons are slightly brown.
8. When done, let them sit for a few minutes to harden as they cool.

13. Cast Iron Deep Dish Cauliflower Crust

Prep Time: 20 Minutes

Cook Time: 40 Minutes

Servings: 5 Slices

Ingredients

- 4 cups cauliflower rice

- 2 eggs

- 1/3 cup almond flour

- 1/3 cup panko crumbs

- Salt and pepper to taste

Instructions

1. First preheat your oven to 425 degrees.
2. Steam and release the moisture from the cauliflower rice. I bought the rice pre-made as I think it is easier and less

time consuming! You can either steam the cauliflower in a pot of water over medium to high heat for about 7 minutes OR place in a microwaveable safe dish and place in the microwave for about 4-5 minutes. Then, allow to cool for a few minutes and place the rice into a paper towel or clean dish cloth and squeeze out any excess moisture.

3. In a large bowl add ALL of the ingredients and mix until well combined.

4. Place your cast iron pan on medium to high heat and add about 2-3 tbsp. of olive oil. Allow to heat for about 1-2 minutes.

5. Add the cauliflower "dough" into the cast iron pan and then press down firmly using a large spoon or spatula!

6. Allow to cook over the stove top for about 10 minutes on medium heat.

7. While the cauliflower crust is cooking – I scrapped the edges a bit so they were completely stuck to the side of the cast iron pan.

8. After 10 minutes, place the cast iron into the oven and bake at 425 degrees for 20 minutes.

9. After 20 minutes, leaving the oven on, add your toppings to the crust.

10. Bake for another 10 minutes or so. For the last few minutes you can turn the oven to broil and allow the top to became a bit crisper!

11. Slice and serve! The first slice may be a bit tricky getting out of the cast iron, so I suggest using a spatula!

12. To reheat simply place under the broiler for about 3 minutes! Lasts up to one week in the fridge.

14. Honey Mustard Asparagus Bacon Salad

Prep Time: 15 minutes

Cook Time: 25 minutes

Servings: 1

Ingredients

For the salad:

- 1-2 pieces of bacon – chopped into bits and cooked until crispy
- 1 hard-boiled egg – cut in half
- 5 spears asparagus – chopped into 1 inch pieces
- 2 mushrooms – sliced into thin pieces
- 2 large handfuls of spinach
- For the dressing:
- 2 tablespoons Dijon mustard
- 1 tablespoon raw local honey
- 1 teaspoon avocado or extra virgin olive oil

Instructions

1. Cook your bacon bits over medium heat in a medium sized skillet on the stove. The bacon will sizzle and crackle and make your whole house smell like breakfast. Cook it until it is crispy and then place it on a paper towel lined plate to soak up the grease.
2. Hard-boil your egg(s). We follow Betty Crocker for the best hard-boiled eggs. Place your eggs in a medium sized saucepan. Cover with cold water at least 1 inch above the egg(s). Heat to a boil in your saucepan; remove from heat. Cover and let stand for 18 minutes.
3. Immediately cool briefly in cold water to prevent further cooking. Tap egg to crack shell; roll between hands to loosen the shell, then peel. If the shell is hard to peel, hold the egg under cold water while peeling.
4. On a salad plate, layer your spinach, mushrooms, asparagus, bacon and hard-boiled egg(s).
5. Drizzle your salad with your honey mustard dressing and eat up! The hard-boiled egg adds protein to your salad so you've got a complete meal. You could also add some grilled or baked chicken or salmon on top for more good fats!

15. Mozzarella Parmesan Stuffed Chicken

Prep Time: 10 Minutes

Cook Time: 20 Minutes

Servings: 2

Ingredients

- 2 large organic chicken breasts

- 2 cups chopped kale

- 1/3 cup shredded mozzarella

- 1/3 cup grated parmesan

- 1/2 teaspoon salt

- 1/4 teaspoon pepper

- 1/4 teaspoon garlic powder

- Spritz of fresh lemon juice

Instructions

1. Preheat oven to 350.
2. Start by cooking down the kale greens. Spray a cast iron skillet with non-stick cooking spray and turn the burner

to medium/low heat. Add the greens along with a dash of salt and cook until tender. This will take about 5 minutes.

3. Remove the greens from the skillet to cool.

4. In a small bowl, toss the cheeses with the kale. Set aside.

5. Lay the chicken on a clean surface.

6. Place the palm of your hand on top of the chicken breast and make a 2-3″ slit in the thickest part of the breast, making sure not to cut all the way through. You want to make a pocket for the cheese and kale mixture. Do this with both chicken breasts.

7. Stuff the cheese and kale mixture into the pocket of the chicken.

8. Season the chicken on both sides with salt, pepper, and garlic powder.

9. In a cast iron skillet, add the olive oil and butter. Melt over medium/high heat.

10. Once the butter has melted, carefully add the chicken breasts to the skillet.

11. Cook on the first side for about 3-4 minutes. Turn the burner to medium if it gets too hot.

12. After it cooks on the first side, flip to the second side and cook for another 3 minutes.

13. After the 3 minutes, cook in the oven for a final 8-10 minutes.

14. Remove from the oven and let the chicken rest.

15. Squeeze fresh lemon juice over top while still warm.

16. Stir-fried Rice Noodles with Ginger Beef

Prep Time: 5 minutes

Cook Time: 15 minutes

Servings: 4

Ingredients

- 1 tablespoon canola oil

- 1 large onion (chopped)

- 3 cups broccoli florets

- 1 cup shredded carrots

- 1 package of Gardein Beefless Tips

- 1 tablespoon fresh garlic (minced)

- 1 teaspoon ground ginger

- 2 tablespoons rice vinegar

- 1 tablespoon sherry cooking wine

- 1 tablespoon soy sauce

- 2 tablespoons water

- ¾ cup low-sodium vegetable broth

- 2 tablespoons unbleached flour

- 2 cups cooked rice noodles

- 2 tablespoons sesame oil

- ¼ cup unsalted peanuts, if desired for garnishing

Instructions

1. Place canola oil in a large wok over high heat, and add chopped onion. Cook for 5 minutes.

2. Add broccoli florets to wok, and cook for 3 minutes before adding shredded carrots, Gardein Beefless tips, minced garlic, and ground ginger.

3. Reduce heat to medium, and cover the wok with a lid to steam the vegetables before continuing to cook.

4. In a separate bowl, stir together rice vinegar, sherry cooking wine, soy sauce, water, vegetable broth, and flour to make a stir-fry sauce.

5. Pour stir fry sauce into the wok, and continue to cook on medium heat until sauce thickens.

6. Add cooked rice noodles to the wok, and stir to coat with sauce and vegetables.

7. Divide evenly onto 3-4 plates, and sprinkle with crushed peanuts to garnish before serving.

17. Curry Roasted Vegetable Quinoa Bowl

Prep Time: 30

Cook Time: 15

Servings: 4

Ingredients

- 1 cup quinoa
- 2 cups vegetable broth
- 1 small head cauliflower, cut into florets
- 1 sweet potato, ½" dice
- 2 cups Brussel sprouts, bottoms trimmed and cut into quarters
- 3 tablespoons coconut oil
- 1 teaspoon curry powder
- 1/2 teaspoon turmeric or Superfood Turmeric
- 1/2 teaspoon cumin
- 1/2 teaspoon sea salt
- ¼ teaspoon black pepper
- 1/4 teaspoon smoked paprika
- 4 cups kale, washed and cut into bite-sized pieces
- 1 ripe avocado, cut into slices

For The Dressing

- 1 ounce lemon juice
- 2 ounces coconut oil
- Sea Salt
- Pepper

Instructions

1. Preheat oven to 375.
2. Place cauliflower, sweet potatoes and brussel sprouts on a baking sheet.
3. Whisk together 3 tablespoons coconut oil, curry powder, turmeric, cumin, salt, pepper and paprika.
4. Pour mixture over the veggies and toss to combine. Roast on the center rack for 20 to 30 minutes, flipping halfway through.
5. While the veggies are roasting, add quinoa and vegetable broth to a small saucepan.
6. Bring to a boil, cover and reduce to simmer for 15 minutes.
7. Remove from heat and package.
8. Sauté kale in coconut oil and season with salt and pepper.
9. Whisk together the dressing ingredients.

10. To serve, place quinoa on the bottom, then a layer of kale, then the roasted veggies and top with the avocado slices and dressing.

Prep Time: 15

Cook Time: 50 minutes

Total Time: 1 hour 5 minutes

Servings: 2

Ingredients

- 1 tilapia filet (use any white fish you like, 1 filet per person)
- 1 tablespoons of Chile Lime Seasoning
- 1/2 cup Coconut Flour (optional, could use other flour or none at all)
- 1 egg, beaten
- 2 small sweet potatoes or 1 large per person, diced
- 1/2 yellow or sweet onion, diced
- 1 tablespoons of onion salt, for the potatoes
- 1/2 bag of butter lettuce
- 1/2 an avocado
- 1 cup of pico de gallo

- 2 tablespoons of salsa verde

Instructions

1. Cut your sweet potato into little bite sized pieces, toss in olive oil and the onion salt seasoning and roast in the oven at 400F for 30-35 minutes.

2. Remove from the oven and finish sautéing in a pan with the diced onion until it's all fully cooked about 5 minutes

3. Put your coconut flour on a plate or shallow bowl with the chile lime seasoning mixed in.
4. Beat the egg in a shallow wide bowl.
5. Rinse and pat dry your fish, then dredge in the coconut flour/seasoning mix covering all sides, give it a quick egg bath, and then once more in the flour mixture
6. Pan sear the fish on high heat in your choice of oil until golden on both sides about 5 minuntes total, then place in the oven at 400 for 10 minutes or until done.
7. Fill a shallow bowl with butter lettuce, add a few big spoonfuls of pico de gallo, then sprinkle liberally with

your sweet potatoes, add the sliced avocado and tilapia.

8. Top the whole thing with salsa verde for extra flavor and brightness!

19. Cinnamon Butternut Squash with Chickpeas

Prep Time: 10 minutes

Cook Time: 30 minutes

Total Time: 40 minutes

Servings: 6

Ingredients

- cups butternut squash- peeled, seeded & chopped into cubes.
- 1 garlic clove, crushed
- 2 tablespoons olive oil
- 3 teaspoons cinnamon
- 2 7 oz can chickpeas, drained
- ½ red onion, thinly sliced
- 1 large bunch coriander, roughly chopped
- Steamed spinach to serve
- Ground black pepper

For the tahini dressing

- 1 garlic clove, crushed
- 3 tablespoons tahini paste

- Juice of 1 lemon

Instructions

1. Preheat oven to 400 F.

2. Toss the squash in the olive oil and season with the crushed garlic and cinnamon. Place in a roasting tin and roast till soft.

3. Place in a roasting tin and roast till soft.

4. Meanwhile rinse and drain the chickpeas and pour them chickpeas into a saucepan with 1/2 cup water. Bring to the boil over a medium heat. Cook to soften slightly and warm through. Bring the water and chickpeas to the boil over a medium heat. Cook to soften slightly and warm through.

5. While the chickpeas are simmering add spinach to a pan with water and wilt for 2-3mins.

6. Drain and set aside the chickpeas.

7. In a large bowl gently toss the butternut squash, chickpeas, wilted spinach, onion and coriander. Add black pepper to season and tahini dressing to taste.

8. Tahini dressing

9. In a bowl add the tahini paste, crushed garlic and lemon juice.

10. Use a fork to whisk and mix well and add up to 5 tablespoons of cold water as you go along.

11. Whisk until the consistency of the dressing is somewhere between single and double cream.

20. Lentil Shepherds Pie

Prep Time: 20 minutes

Cook Time: 50 minutes

Total Time: 1 hour 10 minutes

Servings: 8

Ingredients

- 2 tablespoons olive oil
- 1 medium sweet white onion, finely chopped
- 3 cloves of garlic, pressed or finely chopped
- 2 tablespoons dried basil
- 1 tablespoons dried oregano
- 1 teaspoon cumin
- 1/2 teaspoon cinnamon
- 1/4 teaspoon cloves
- season to taste – this may be best to do at the end!
- 3/4 cup tomato puree
- 2 heaped teaspoon tomato paste
- 2 tablespoons vegetable stock paste
- 1 1/2 cups cooked lentils – I used Bob's Red Mill

- 1 packet Yves Ground Round
- 2-3 cups hot water
- season to taste
- 5 large white potatoes, peeled and cubed
- season to taste
- 1 tablespoon olive oil
- 1/4 – 1/2 cup almond milk
- 1 heaped tablespoons butter
- 1 teaspoon fresh thyme
- garnish with 2 tablespoons fresh thyme

Instructions

1. Into a large pot add olive oil and heat for 30 seconds on medium-high heat. Add your onions and cook for around 5 minutes or until soft and translucent. Add in your garlic, basil, oregano, cumin, cinnamon and cloves. Stir until onion is well coated and turn heat to low to cook and marry for around 3 minutes. Stir often to avoid burning.

2. Into the pot add your tomato puree, tomato paste and vegetable stock paste. Give this all a good stir and then increase heat to high before adding your lentils and Yves Ground Round. Let them sautéed in the pan

for two minutes before adding your water. Stir, stir, stir, bring to a boil then simmer for 20 minutes until thick and luscious like a traditional meat sauce. Set aside once done.

3. Preheat oven to 400F and line a baking sheet with parchment paper.

4. While your "meat" sauce is simmering prepare your mashed potatoes by boiling water in a large stockpot. Season your water and cook your potatoes till very tender, could take 15 minutes or so. Strain your potatoes but absolutely do not rinse and return to pot. Add the remainder of the ingredients and mash till extremely rich and creamy! Remember, when adding your liquid that you must have a more solid mash to add on top of the first layer! Set aside.

5. Into a 13"L x 7.75"W x 2.25"H baking dish transfer your "meat mixture" and lay it flat using a spatula. Begin dolloping your mashed potato onto the mixture and using a flat tool flatten it all out. I like using a fork to carve marks vertically and horizontally across the pie. This adds fun texture and when it cooks gets nice and golden brown! Before cooking spray the mashed potatoes with an oil of your choice for that

added golden colour (you will thank me later if you do this).

6. Cook for 25 minutes before setting the oven to broil for 5 minutes. Watch closely so nothing burns but this is an amazing adding touch to the recipe!

7. Enjoy with fresh thyme garnish and your choice of steamed greens or veg!

DINNER

21. Braised Turkey Thighs with Winter Roots
Prep Time: 30 minutes

Cook Time: 2 hours

Total Time: 2 hours 30 minutes

Servings: 2

Ingredients

- 2 pastured turkey thighs (season with sea salt, black pepper, cumin and cayenne)
- 3-4 tablespoons peanut oil (or other high smoke point oil; coconut, lard, schmaltz)
- 3 cups water (turkey stock or chicken stock)
- 3 cups white wine
- 1 bay leaf
- 1 teaspoon dried rosemary
- 2 teaspoons dried sage
- 1 teaspoon dried thyme
- 1 onion (peeled and chopped)

- 2-3 carrots (chopped)
- 1 rutabaga (cut into 1 inch pieces)
- 4 garlic cloves (peeled and minced)
- 1 teaspoon real salt
- black pepper to taste
- parsley

Instructions

1. Put fat/oil into a deep frying pan on medium heat. When oil begins shimmering (getting wavy), put two turkey thighs into the pan and lightly brown on each side (4-5 minutes). Discard excess oil.

2. Add water, wine, and bay leaf into the pan with the seared turkey thighs and bring to a boil. Cover and lower heat to simmer for 1 hour and 15 minutes.

3. Turn turkey thighs at least one time during that cooking time. Add herbs, onions, carrots, rutabaga and garlic, plus sea salt and black pepper. Adjust salt and pepper to taste.

4. Cover and continue cooking until almost all the liquid is gone (45 minutes). Save some liquid to use for gravy.

5. Plate braised turkey and winter roots. Spoon a little gravy from the pan and garnish with fresh parsley.

22. Sesame Tamari Brussels Sprouts

Prep Time: 10 minutes

Cook Time: 35 Minutes

Total Time: 45 minutes

Servings: 4

Ingredients

- 1/12 pound brussels sprouts (stems cut, outer layer removed and halved lengthwise)
- 1 Japanese sweet potato (half moon chopped, yams work too)
- ¼ cup sesame oil
- ¼ cup rice vinegar
- ¼ cup tamari (or soy sauce)
- 1 tablespoon maple syrup
- 2 cups red seedless grapes (halved)
- ½ cup roasted peanuts

Instructions

1. 1Preheat oven to 400F.

2. 2 Place Brussels Sprouts in a large bowl.

3. 3 Whisk the tamari, sesame oil, maple syrup and rice vinegar together then pour over the sprouts. Make sure to coat the sprouts evenly.

4. 4 Line a baking tray with parchment paper. Place the sprouts cut side down on the tray. Pour any remaining dressing over the sprouts.

5. 5 Roast for 35-ish minutes (the sesame roasting smell will make your house smell like you know what you're doing in the kitchen). You want the sprouts to be charred and crispy.

6. 6Place the grapes and nuts in a bowl. Add the still hot Brussels Sprouts. Mix that up, and you're done.

23. BBQ Tempeh and Pineapple Skewers

Prep Time: 30 Mintes

Cook Time: 12 Minutes

Total   Time: 42 minutes

Servings: 4

Ingredients

- 1 package of tempeh

- 1 bottle of your favorite BBQ sauce (check the label to keep it gluten-free)

- 2 cups pineapple

- 2 bell peppers

- 1 large zucchini

- 1 small red onion

- 2 tablespoons avocado or olive oil

- wooden skewers

Instructions

1. To prep the tempeh: start by slicing the block into large pieces and add to a large freezer bag or container.

2. Pour in about 1/2 cup of the BBQ sauce and toss to coat the tempeh. Place in the fridge for 30 minutes to marinate while you prep the other ingredients.

3. To prep the grain: if serving with a grain, boil the water and cook the as directed on the package. Cover and set aside when ready to keep warm.

4. To prep the veggies: wash and slice all of the remaining veggies and pineapple into large bite-sized pieces (you want them big enough that they won't break/fall off the skewers.

5. Warm up the grill or grill pan on medium-high heat.

6. To assemble the skewers: lightly wet the wooden skewers to prevent them from burning. Slide, in any order, the marinated tempeh, pineapple, and veggies onto a skewer leaving enough empty space at each end to pick it up. Place it on a dish and continue until all of the ingredients are used up. Brush each skewer with a little oil to prevent sticking to the grill.

7. To cook: place the skewers on the preheated grill or grill pan. You want a nice sear so you should hear a sizzle once the skewers are over the heat. Cook for about 5 minutes

and rotate. Continue rotating every 5 minutes until each side has been seared and the veggies are just slightly tender.

8. Serve warm over the grain with a side of BBQ for dipping!

24. Tuna Sashimi with Avocado Salad

Prep Time:10 minutes

Cook Time: N/a

Servings: 2

Ingredients

- 1 tablespoon olive oil
- 1/2 teaspoon sesame oil
- 1 tablespoon tamari
- 1 tablespoon rice vinegar
- a dash of wasabi
- 175 g fillet of fresh tuna, cut into thin slices

FOR THE SALAD

- 1 avocado, sliced
- 8 cherry tomatoes, halved
- 2 heaped tablespoons freshly torn cilantro
- 3 spring onions, sliced
- juice of 1 lime
- sea salt and freshly ground black pepper
- 1 teaspoon toasted sesame seeds as garnish

Instructions

1. Pour the olive oil, sesame oil, tamari sauce and rice vinegar into a dish, then whisk in the wasabi. Add the tuna and coat well.
2. Layer the avocado, tomatoes, coriander and spring onions, squeeze over the lime juice and season to taste. Top with the dressed tuna and a sprinkling of sesame seeds.

25. Chunky Sweet Potato and Sweet Pepper Soup (Vegan)

Prep Time: 5 minutes

Cook Time: 45 minutes

Total   Time: 50 minutes

Servings: 6

Ingredients

- 1 tablespoon olive oil
- 1 red onion, chopped
- 4 celery stalks, diced
- 4 carrots, chopped
- 5 garlic cloves, minced
- 1 tablespoon coriander seeds
- 1/4 teaspoon crushed red pepper
- stems of a basil bunch, chopped
- 3 sweet potatoes, chopped
- 3 portobello mushrooms, chopped
- 4 bell peppers, chopped
- 2 15 ounce cans of chickpeas
- 10 cups water
- 2 vegetable bullion cubes

- salt and pepper to taste
- 1/4 cup pepitas, toasted
- a handful of fresh basil, chiffonade

Instructions

1. In a large soup pot, heat the olive oil over medium-high heat. Add the onion, carrots, and celery. Saute for 3 minutes.
2. Add the bell pepper, portobello mushrooms, garlic, chopped basil stems, coriander seeds, and crushed red pepper. Saute for 2 minutes.
3. Add the sweet potato, water, and vegetable bullion. Bring to a boil and reduce to a simmer. In a bowl, mash 1 can of the chickpeas and leave the other can whole. Add to the soup.
4. When the sweet potatoes are cooked through, add the chopped kale and season taste with salt and pepper.
5. Serve in warmed bowls and garnish with toasted pepitas and fresh basil.

Prep Time: 5 Minutes

Cook Time: 25 Minutes

Total   Time: 30 minutes

Servings: 6

Ingredients

Soup:

- 1-2 lbs chicken breast

- ¼ onion

- 5 small-medium organic Yukon gold potatoes

- 3 carrots (about 1 cup chopped)

- 1 cup frozen peas

- 1 bag frozen cauliflower

- 1 tablespoon ghee

- 1 tablespoon avocado oil or olive oil

- 3 cups chicken bone broth or chicken broth

- 1 cup almond milk

- 1 cup coconut milk

- 1 tablespoon garlic powder

- 1 tablespoon onion powder

- 2 tablespoon salt

- ½ tablespoon pepper

- 1 tablespoon thyme

- Crust Crumbles:
- 1 cup almond four

- 1 egg

- ½ tablespoon ghee, melted

- ½ tablespoon garlic powder

- Pinch sea salt

Instructions

1. Preheat oven to 400° for your crumbles.
2. Cube and cook chicken in avocado oil/olive oil. While cooking, chop veggies and begin to cook in the bottom of a pot with ghee.

3. After a few minutes, add in bone broth/chicken broth, almond milk and coconut milk. Cook until the potatoes are fork tender.

4. Remove three cups of broth and veggies from the pot and blend until completely smooth. This is great way to thicken soups without adding flours!

5. Add the blended mixture and the chicken back to the pot. Let sit on med-low while preparing the crumbles.

6. Combine almond flour, garlic power, salt, melted ghee and an egg and stir until perfectly mixed.

7. Line a cookie sheet with parchment paper and crumble apart the dough until little "crumbles" fill the sheet. Bake for 10-12 minutes until slightly golden.

8. Serve soup warm with the crumbles on top and enjoy!

Prep Time: 5-10 minutes

Cook Time :20 minutes

Servings :4

Ingredients

- 3/4 cup cooked wild rice (mixture of black, red, brown rice)

- Vegetable Mixture
- 1/2 red onion, diced
- 2-3 cloves of garlic, minced
- 1 1/2 cups of broccoli or broccolini, chopped
- 2/3 cup of mushroom (choose between or use mixture of crimini, shiitake, oyster, maitake), chopped
- 1/2 red pepper, chopped (optional)
- 2 tablespoons butter and avocado oil
- Cheese Sauce
- 2 tablespoons butter
- 1cup whole milk
- 2 tablespoons flour
- 1 teaspoon dijon mustard
- Pinch of cayenne pepper

- 8-12 ounces grated Parmesan Reggiano cheese or cheddar cheese

Instructions

1. Heat oven to 400 degrees

2. Heat 1 tbsp butter and 1 tbsp avocado oil in a cast iron over medium heat. Once melted, add onion and saute until translucent, about 5 minutes.

3. Then slowly add in your chopped broccoli, mushrooms, garlic, and red pepper if using. Sprinkle in salt and pepper and saute until cooked through and then remove from heat.

4. To make the cheese sauce, in a small pan melt 2 tbsp butter over low heat. Once melted, add flour and whisk until combined. Slowly drizzle in milk, whisking constantly, until sauce is slightly thickened, about 2 minutes.

5. Remove pan from heat and stir in Dijon mustard and 1/3 of grated cheese. Season generously with salt and pepper.

6. Add cooked rice to your vegetable mixture and mix well. Then pour cheese sauce over and gently mix

to ensure all pieces get some sauce. Sprinkle remaining cheese over top. Bake casserole for 10 to 15 minutes, until the cheese has mostly melted, then run under the broiler until cheese is toasty on top.

28. Sweet Potato and Cranberry Salad

Prep Time: 10 minutes

Cook Time: 25 minutes

Total Time: 35 minutes

Servings: 6

Ingredients

- Sweet Potato & Cranberry Salad
- 2 pounds organic sweet potatoes (about 3 large), peeled & cubed
- 1 small diced red onion
- 2 tablespoon. olive oil
- salt, black pepper & garlic powder
- 1/2 cup dried organic cranberries
- 1/2 cup crumbled feta cheese
- 1/4 cup chopped fresh parsley
- Vinaigrette:
- 2 tablespoons apple cider vinegar
- 1 tablespoon Dijon mustard
- 1 tablespoon maple syrup or raw honey
- 1/2 teaspoon ground cumin
- 1/4 teaspoon smoked paprika
- 1/4 cup olive oil

- salt & pepper, to taste

Instructions

1. Preheat oven to 400. Line a baking sheet with foil or parchment paper. Spread sweet potato and onion out on the baking sheet. Drizzle with olive oil and season with salt, pepper and garlic powder. Toss to evenly coat, making sure to spread potatoes in a single layer if possible. Put in the oven for 20-25 minutes (or until fork-tender), tossing once or twice.

2. Meanwhile, make the dressing by combing all ingredients in a small jar or bottle with a lid (I'm a HUGE fan of using mason jars to make salad dressing). Shake until well-blended and taste for seasoning.

3. Once sweet potatoes are cooked, place in a large bowl and allow to cool. Once they're cool, add in cranberries, feta, and parsley, stirring gently to mix.

4. When you're ready to serve the salad, add a little at a time, again tossing gently to distribute. I had a little dressing leftover, but it's a matter of preference how much you use.

5. This salad can be served slightly warm or tastes just as good chilled.

29. Marinated Pork Tenderloin Traybake

Prep Time: 15 minutes

Cook Time: 30 - 40 minutes

Servings: 2

Ingredients

- 1 pork tenderloin fillet (enough to feed two people)
- 2 parsnips (peeled and quartered)
- 2 carrots (peeled and quartered)
- handful of potatoes (cut into bitesize pieces, with the skin on)
- 1 large bramely apple (peeled and cut into cubes-leave out if following FODMAP diet)
- 1 large red onion (cut into wedges- again, leave out if following FODMAP diet)
- 1 tablespoon dijon mustard
- 1 teaspoon each of dried rosemary, sage and thyme
- salt and pepper
- 1 tablespoon oil
- optional: Your choice of greens to serve

Instructions

1. Preheat the oven to 190 degrees F.

2. Place all the vegetables into a tray, drizzle with the oil, salt, pepper, and half the herbs. Place in the oven and cook for 10 minutes.

3. Take the pork tenderloin fillet and spread over the dijon mustard, then roll in the herbs and salt and pepper until coated.

4. Take the tray of veg out the oven, mix, then place the pork tenderloin on top of the vegetables. Cook for 30 – 40 minutes until the pork is cooked through, although I like to leave mine slightly pink in the middle so it doesn't dry out.

5. Take the pork out and leave to rest on a board for 10 minutes before slicing, serving on top of the roasted vegetables.

30. Cauliflower Fried Rice (High Fiber, Vegan)

Prep Time: 5 minutes

Cook Time: 10 minutes

Total Time: 15 minutes

Servings: 4

Ingredients

- 1 bag of frozen cauliflower rice
- 1 cup frozen/fresh corn
- 1 cup frozen shelled edamame
- 1 cup chopped rainbow carrots (or regular carrots will do)
- about 1/4 cup diced onion
- 1-2 cloves minced garlic
- 1 tablespoon olive oil
- 2 teaspoon Thai chili paste/sauce
- 1- 1.5 tablespoon low sodium soy sauce
- 1 teaspoon toasted sesame oil

Instructions

1. Start by heating the oil in a pan over medium heat. Add in the garlic and onion and cook until golden
2. Meanwhile, prepare all of the vegetables. Add all the veggies to the pan except the cauliflower rice. Cover and cook for about 5 minutes until they start to tenderize.
3. Add the cauliflower, chilli paste, soy sauce & sesame oil and stir until well mixed. Cover & cook for another 5 minutes stirring often!
4. Serve however you desire! I served mine over a bed of kale!

SNACKS

Prep Time: 30-40 minutes

Cook Time: N/A

Servings: 36

Ingredients

- 1/2 cup coconut oil
- 1/2 cup cocoa butter
- 4 tablespoons cashew butter (or any nut butter of your choice)
- 1 teaspoon Further Food Superfood Turmeric
- 1/2 teaspoon vanilla
- 1/8 teaspoon Himalayan pink sea salt
- 4 tablespoons unsweetened pumpkin

Instructions

1. Combine all ingredients and melt it into a pan over stovetop.
2. Whisk while heating to blend it up and then pour into your favorite molds.

3. Refrigerate molds for 30 minutes

32. Dried Plum and Pistachio Chia Pudding

Prep Time: 5 minutes

Cook Time: 60 minutes (to chill and set)

Servings:b2

Ingredients

- 1/3 cup chia seeds
- 1 1/2 cups unsweetened almond milk (or other non-dairy milk)
- 1/2 cup California Dried Plums (chopped) + additional for topping
- 1/3 cup pistachios roasted + additional for topping
- 2 tablespoons hemp seeds
- 1 tablespoon cacao nibs unsweetened + additional for topping
- 2 teaspoon cinnamon ground

Instructions

1. Whisk together ingredients in large mixing bowl.

2. Cover and chill in fridge for at least one hour or overnight.

3. Once mixture reaches a pudding-like consistency, remove from fridge and divide into 2 bowls or mason jars.

4. Top with additional chopped California Dried Plums, pistachios, and cacao nibs before serving.

33. Quick & Easy Tahini Cookies

Prep Time: 10 Minutes

Cook Time: 8-12 Minutes

Servings: 11

Ingredients

- 1 cup drippy tahini
- 1/2 cup coconut sugar
- 1 pasture-raised egg
- 1 teaspoon pure vanilla extract
- 1/2 cup sugar-free dark chocolate chips

Instructions

1. Preheat oven to 350°F and line a cookie tray with parchment.
2. Put tahini, sweetener, egg, and vanilla into a large bowl. Beat together until smooth. Fold in chocolate chips.
3. Roll dough into 10 to 12 balls. Place on tray (I used 2 trays to spread them out more) and press down gently with a fork.

4. Bake for 8-12 min, until just golden brown around the edges (see note below*). As soon as they come out of the oven, sprinkle top with some sea salt flakes if desired.

5. Allow cookies to cool on the baking sheet for 10 minutes, then transfer to a wire rack to finish cooling.

34. Peanut Butter Cookies with Caramel Drizzle

Prep Time: 10 Minutes

Cook Time: 30 Minutes

Total Time: 40 minutes

Servings: 15 Cookies

Ingredients

Peanut Butter Cookies:

- 1 cup unsweetened natural peanut butter

- 1/2 cup almond flour

- 3 tablespoon coconut flour

- 2 eggs

- 1/2 cup raw organic honey

- 1 teaspoon pure vanilla extract

- 1/2 teaspoon baking soda

- 1/4 teaspoon salt

- 1 teaspoon cinnamon

Caramel:

- 1 cup canned coconut milk, full fat

- 1 tablespoon coconut oil

- 1/2 cup raw organic honey

- 1 teaspoon pure vanilla extract

- 1/2 teaspoon sea salt

Instructions

1. Get your caramel sauce started first by combining the coconut milk, coconut oil, honey and vanilla extract in a sauce pan over medium-high heat.
2. Bring to a boil, but keeping a close eye as it can quickly boil over, then immediately lower the temperature, keeping the caramel sauce at a light simmer. Simmer for about 25-30 minutes, stirring occasionally.
3. Preheat oven to 350F degrees.
4. In a food processor, combine all of your cookie ingredients together until the dough starts to form a ball.
5. Line a baking sheet with parchment paper and place one-inch balls evenly apart.
6. Flatten each ball with the back of a fork slightly to make the lines in the middle.
7. Bake for about 10-12 minutes and cool for 5 minutes.
8. Drizzle caramel sauce over cookie and indulge!

35. Easy Keto Cheesy Biscuits

Prep Time: 10 minutes

Cook Time: 15 minutes

Total Time: 25 minutes

Servings: 8-10

Ingredients

- 9 ounces almond flour
- ½ teaspoon salt
- 4 teaspoons baking powder
- 1 tablespoon konjac flour / glucomannan powder
- 2 tablespoons gelatin such as Further Food Premium Gelatin
- 2 ounces cold butter, cut into small pieces
- 2 ½ ounces sharp (strong) cheddar cheese, finely grated
- 1 egg
- 2 tablespoons unsweetened coconut milk (carton) or any unsweetened nut milk
- 1 beaten egg to glaze

Instructions

1. Heat oven to 375 F.
2. Put the almond flour, other dry ingredients and butter in a food processor and pulse until it resembles fine breadcrumbs. You can also do this by hand if that's your thing.
3. Turn into a bowl and mix in the cheese until evenly distributed.
4. In a cup or small bowl, whisk the egg and nut milk together well.
5. Make a well in the center of the dry ingredients and pour in the egg / nut milk liquid.
6. Quickly mix by hand to form a dough.
7. Knead the dough lightly until smooth.
8. Roll out the dough to ¾ inch thick, or thicker if you like. Especially if you're going to use them as sandwich biscuits.
9. Cut out biscuits using a round or fluted cutter, or cut them into squares with a sharp knife.
10. Gather up the trimmings into a ball, re-roll and cut remaining dough into biscuits.
11. Place the scones on a baking sheet lined with parchment paper.
12. Brush tops with a beaten egg.

13. Bake for 15 – 17 minutes until golden brown.

Prep Time: 10 minutes

Cook Time: 15 minutes

Total Time: 25 minutes

Servings: 23 Balls

Ingredients

- ½ cup almonds
- ½ cup cashews
- ½ cup coconut
- 2 limes, juiced
- 1 tablespoon lime zest (from about 2 limes)
- 9 dates, soaked & pitted
- ⅛ tsp salt

Instructions

1. Place the almonds, cashews and coconut in a food processor and pulse until they're finely ground.

2. Add the remaining ingredients and pulse again until smooth.

3. Take 1 tablespoon of mixture and roll it into a ball.

4. Place on a tray that's been lined with parchment. Repeat with the remaining mixture until all balls are formed.

5. Sprinkle extra lime zest over the tops of each ball before storing.

6. If rolling in coconut: Pour coconut shreds in a bowl. Take one ball and roll it in the coconut until all the times are covered. Set aside. Repeat with remaining balls.

37. Honey Mustard Cheddar Chicken Meatballs

Prep Time: 5 minutes

Cook Time: 20 minutes

Total Time: 25 minutes

Servings: 4

Ingredients

Meatballs:

- 1 pound ground chicken, 93% or 98% lean or ground turkey
- 1/4 cup quick-cooking oats
- 1/4 cup cheddar cheese
- 1 clove minced garlic
- 1/2 teaspoon onion powder
- 1/2 teaspoon parsley
- 1/2 teaspoon sea salt
- 1/4 teaspoon freshly ground black pepper

Honey Mustard Dressing:

- 4 tablespoons yellow mustard
- 4 tablespoons organic honey
- 1/8-1/4 teaspoon chili powder or paprika

Instructions

1. Preheat oven to 400 degrees.
2. Mix all of the ingredients for the chicken meatballs in a large mixing bowl.
3. Mix all of the ingredients for the honey mustard in a separate bowl.
4. Reserve half of the dressing.
5. Roll the chicken mixture into 1-1.5″ balls. Place on a lined or non-stick baking sheet sprayed with a little cooking oil.
6. Top each meatball with some of the honey mustard dressing.
7. Bake for 20-23 minutes.
8. Take out of the oven and top with more of the dressing. Ready to eat!

38. Pecan Pie Baked Collagen Oatmeal

Prep Time: 10 minutes

Cook Time: 25 minutes

Total Time: 35 minutes

Servings: 8

Ingredients

- 2 cups rolled oats
- 2 eggs
- 3 tablespoons coconut sugar
- 1 teaspoon cinnamon
- 1 teaspoon vanilla
- pinch of salt
- 1 1/2 cup almond milk
- 4 scoops Further Food Collagen Protein Peptides
- 3 tablespoons grass fed butter – melted

Toppings:
- 1/4 cups pecans
- 1/4 cups maple syrup

Instructions

1. Preheat oven to 375 degrees.

2. Add dry ingredients to a large bowl (Oats, coconut sugar, cinnamon, salt, collagen) and stir until combined.

3. Add wet ingredients into another bowl (eggs, vanilla, almond milk, butter) and whisk until combined.

4. Add wet ingredients to dry ingredients and fold together until well combined.

5. Add mixture to a greased baking dish. You can grease with butter, coconut oil or cooking spray.

6. Smooth mixture into dish until even and add the pecans.

7. Put dish in oven for 15 minutes.

8. Take out and add the maple syrup.

9. Put back in oven and bake for an additional 10 minutes.

10. Take out, let cool and enjoy. Cut into squares and store in an air tight container in the fridge for up to a week and a half.

Prep Time: 10 Minutes

Cook Time: 13 Minutes

Total Time: 23 minutes

Servings: 24 Bites

Ingredients

- ½ cup cranberry sauce (store bought or homemade)

- 4 oz. brie cheese wheel

- 1 8oz. package crescent roll dough

- Fresh rosemary sprigs (optional)

Instructions

1. Preheat your oven to 375 degrees and spray a mini muffin with non-stick cooking spray. Place the brie wheel in your freezer for 10-15 minutes while you prepare the dough.

2. Lightly flour a work surface and lay your crescent dough out on the surface. Lightly flour a rolling pin

and roll the dough into a large thin rectangle. Cut the dough into 24 small squares. (Sometimes I'm only able to make 22 squares depending on the shape of my dough.) Place one square into each mini muffin tin.

3. Take the brie out of the freezer and cut it into small cubes (they should be between ½ – ¾ inches on each side). Place 1 cheese cube in the center of each dough square. Spoon 1 teaspoon of your cranberry sauce over top of the brie. Place the muffin tin in the oven and bake for 10-13 minutes or until the dough is golden brown.

4. Once done, let the bites cool for a few minutes before taking them out of the tin. Top each bite with fresh rosemary and chopped nuts (if using) and serve immediately.

40. Ultra Fudgy Freezer Brownies

Prep Time:10 minutes (+1 hour freezing time)

Cook Time: N/A

Servings: 10

Ingredients

- 20 plump Medjool dates
- 1/4 cup of raw cacao powder
- 2 scoops of Further Food Chocolate Collagen
- 1/4 cup creamy almond butter

Instructions

1. In a food processor, add 20 plump Medjool dates, 1/4 cup raw cacao powder, 2 scoops furtherfood chocolate collagen with reishi, 1/4 cup creamy almond butter and blend until you have a smooth batter.
2. Pour into a parchment paper-lined pan and top with raw walnuts.

3. Freeze for 1 hour or until firm, cut into squares, and enjoy.

4. Store in freezer.